D1626960

WINE TASTING NOTES

Personal Details

NAME:

_____

ADDRESS:

_____

_____

PHONE:

_____

E-MAIL:

_____

WINE	PAGE

WINE	PAGE

WINE _____ VINTAGE _____

WHEN _____ WITH _____

WHERE _____ PRICE _____

VARIETAL _____ ALCOHOL (%) _____

BODY   - [| | | | |] +

TANNINS   - [| | | | |] +

SWEETNESS - [| | | | |] +

INTENSITY - [| | | | |] +

FINISH   - [| | | | |] +

SMELL

- [ ] TOAST
- [ ] LEATHER
- [ ] MUSHROOM
- [ ] TOBACCO
- [ ] CHOCOLATE
- [ ] JAM
- [ ]

- [ ] SMOKE
- [ ] COFFEE
- [ ] MINT
- [ ] SPICE
- [ ] PEPPER
- [ ] ALMOND
- [ ]

- [ ] HONEY
- [ ] APPLES
- [ ] GRASS
- [ ] FLORAL
- [ ] TROPICAL
- [ ] VEGETAL
- [ ]

- [ ] MELON
- [ ] CITRUS
- [ ] OAK
- [ ] BERRIES
- [ ] NUTMEG
- [ ]

TASTE

- [ ] NUTMEG
- [ ] VEGETAL
- [ ] FLORAL
- [ ] HONEY
- [ ] PEARS
- [ ] PEACHES
- [ ]

- [ ] EARTH
- [ ] PEPPER
- [ ] VANILLA
- [ ] COFFEE
- [ ] LICORICE
- [ ] LEATHER
- [ ]

- [ ] DARK FRUITS
- [ ] BERRIES
- [ ] PLUMS
- [ ] MUSHROOM
- [ ] TOBACCO
- [ ] CHOCOLATE
- [ ]

- [ ] TOAST
- [ ] GRASS
- [ ] CITRUS
- [ ] MELON
- [ ] LYCHE
- [ ] ALMOND
- [ ]

REVIEW

RATING

WINE _____ VINTAGE _____

WHEN _____ WITH _____

WHERE _____ PRICE _____

VARIETAL _____ ALCOHOL (%) _____

BODY   - [| | | | |] +

TANNINS   - [| | | | |] +

SWEETNESS - [| | | | |] +

INTENSITY - [| | | | |] +

FINISH   - [| | | | |] +

SMELL

☐ TOAST	☐ SMOKE	☐ HONEY	☐ MELON
☐ LEATHER	☐ COFFEE	☐ APPLES	☐ CITRUS
☐ MUSHROOM	☐ MINT	☐ GRASS	☐ OAK
☐ TOBACCO	☐ SPICE	☐ FLORAL	☐ BERRIES
☐ CHOCOLATE	☐ PEPPER	☐ TROPICAL	☐ NUTMEG
☐ JAM	☐ ALMOND	☐ VEGETAL	☐
☐	☐	☐	☐

TASTE

☐ NUTMEG	☐ EARTH	☐ DARK FRUITS	☐ TOAST
☐ VEGETAL	☐ PEPPER	☐ BERRIES	☐ GRASS
☐ FLORAL	☐ VANILLA	☐ PLUMS	☐ CITRUS
☐ HONEY	☐ COFFEE	☐ MUSHROOM	☐ MELON
☐ PEARS	☐ LICORICE	☐ TOBACCO	☐ LYCHE
☐ PEACHES	☐ LEATHER	☐ CHOCOLATE	☐ ALMOND
☐	☐	☐	☐

REVIEW

RATING

WINE _____ VINTAGE _____

WHEN _____ WITH _____

WHERE _____ PRICE _____

VARIETAL _____ ALCOHOL (%) _____

BODY   - | | | | | | | +

TANNINS   - | | | | | | | +

SWEETNESS - | | | | | | | +

INTENSITY - | | | | | | | +

FINISH   - | | | | | | | +

SMELL

- [ ] TOAST
- [ ] LEATHER
- [ ] MUSHROOM
- [ ] TOBACCO
- [ ] CHOCOLATE
- [ ] JAM
- [ ]

- [ ] SMOKE
- [ ] COFFEE
- [ ] MINT
- [ ] SPICE
- [ ] PEPPER
- [ ] ALMOND
- [ ]

- [ ] HONEY
- [ ] APPLES
- [ ] GRASS
- [ ] FLORAL
- [ ] TROPICAL
- [ ] VEGETAL
- [ ]

- [ ] MELON
- [ ] CITRUS
- [ ] OAK
- [ ] BERRIES
- [ ] NUTMEG
- [ ]

TASTE

- [ ] NUTMEG
- [ ] VEGETAL
- [ ] FLORAL
- [ ] HONEY
- [ ] PEARS
- [ ] PEACHES
- [ ]

- [ ] EARTH
- [ ] PEPPER
- [ ] VANILLA
- [ ] COFFEE
- [ ] LICORICE
- [ ] LEATHER
- [ ]

- [ ] DARK FRUITS
- [ ] BERRIES
- [ ] PLUMS
- [ ] MUSHROOM
- [ ] TOBACCO
- [ ] CHOCOLATE
- [ ]

- [ ] TOAST
- [ ] GRASS
- [ ] CITRUS
- [ ] MELON
- [ ] LYCHE
- [ ] ALMOND
- [ ]

REVIEW

RATING

WINE _____ VINTAGE _____

WHEN _____ WITH _____

WHERE _____ PRICE _____

VARIETAL _____ ALCOHOL (%) _____

BODY   - | | | | | | | +

TANNINS   - | | | | | | | +

SWEETNESS - | | | | | | | +

INTENSITY - | | | | | | | +

FINISH   - | | | | | | | +

SMELL

☐ TOAST	☐ SMOKE	☐ HONEY	☐ MELON
☐ LEATHER	☐ COFFEE	☐ APPLES	☐ CITRUS
☐ MUSHROOM	☐ MINT	☐ GRASS	☐ OAK
☐ TOBACCO	☐ SPICE	☐ FLORAL	☐ BERRIES
☐ CHOCOLATE	☐ PEPPER	☐ TROPICAL	☐ NUTMEG
☐ JAM	☐ ALMOND	☐ VEGETAL	☐
☐	☐	☐	☐

TASTE

☐ NUTMEG	☐ EARTH	☐ DARK FRUITS	☐ TOAST
☐ VEGETAL	☐ PEPPER	☐ BERRIES	☐ GRASS
☐ FLORAL	☐ VANILLA	☐ PLUMS	☐ CITRUS
☐ HONEY	☐ COFFEE	☐ MUSHROOM	☐ MELON
☐ PEARS	☐ LICORICE	☐ TOBACCO	☐ LYCHE
☐ PEACHES	☐ LEATHER	☐ CHOCOLATE	☐ ALMOND
☐	☐	☐	☐

REVIEW

RATING

WINE _____ VINTAGE _____

WHEN _____ WITH _____

WHERE _____ PRICE _____

VARIETAL _____ ALCOHOL (%) _____

BODY   - [| | | | |] +

TANNINS   - [| | | | |] +

SWEETNESS   - [| | | | |] +

INTENSITY   - [| | | | |] +

FINISH   - [| | | | |] +

SMELL

☐ TOAST	☐ SMOKE	☐ HONEY	☐ MELON
☐ LEATHER	☐ COFFEE	☐ APPLES	☐ CITRUS
☐ MUSHROOM	☐ MINT	☐ GRASS	☐ OAK
☐ TOBACCO	☐ SPICE	☐ FLORAL	☐ BERRIES
☐ CHOCOLATE	☐ PEPPER	☐ TROPICAL	☐ NUTMEG
☐ JAM	☐ ALMOND	☐ VEGETAL	☐
☐	☐	☐	☐

TASTE

☐ NUTMEG	☐ EARTH	☐ DARK FRUITS	☐ TOAST
☐ VEGETAL	☐ PEPPER	☐ BERRIES	☐ GRASS
☐ FLORAL	☐ VANILLA	☐ PLUMS	☐ CITRUS
☐ HONEY	☐ COFFEE	☐ MUSHROOM	☐ MELON
☐ PEARS	☐ LICORICE	☐ TOBACCO	☐ LYCHE
☐ PEACHES	☐ LEATHER	☐ CHOCOLATE	☐ ALMOND
☐	☐	☐	☐

REVIEW

RATING

WINE _____ VINTAGE _____

WHEN _____ WITH _____

WHERE _____ PRICE _____

VARIETAL _____ ALCOHOL (%) _____

BODY   – | | | | | | | +

TANNINS   – | | | | | | | +

SWEETNESS   – | | | | | | | +

INTENSITY   – | | | | | | | +

FINISH   – | | | | | | | +

SMELL

☐ TOAST	☐ SMOKE	☐ HONEY	☐ MELON
☐ LEATHER	☐ COFFEE	☐ APPLES	☐ CITRUS
☐ MUSHROOM	☐ MINT	☐ GRASS	☐ OAK
☐ TOBACCO	☐ SPICE	☐ FLORAL	☐ BERRIES
☐ CHOCOLATE	☐ PEPPER	☐ TROPICAL	☐ NUTMEG
☐ JAM	☐ ALMOND	☐ VEGETAL	☐
☐	☐	☐	☐

TASTE

☐ NUTMEG	☐ EARTH	☐ DARK FRUITS	☐ TOAST
☐ VEGETAL	☐ PEPPER	☐ BERRIES	☐ GRASS
☐ FLORAL	☐ VANILLA	☐ PLUMS	☐ CITRUS
☐ HONEY	☐ COFFEE	☐ MUSHROOM	☐ MELON
☐ PEARS	☐ LICORICE	☐ TOBACCO	☐ LYCHE
☐ PEACHES	☐ LEATHER	☐ CHOCOLATE	☐ ALMOND
☐	☐	☐	☐

REVIEW

RATING

WINE _____ VINTAGE _____

WHEN _____ WITH _____

WHERE _____ PRICE _____

VARIETAL _____ ALCOHOL (%) _____

BODY   - ☐☐☐☐☐☐ +

TANNINS - ☐☐☐☐☐☐ +

SWEETNESS - ☐☐☐☐☐☐ +

INTENSITY - ☐☐☐☐☐☐ +

FINISH - ☐☐☐☐☐☐ +

SMELL

☐ TOAST	☐ SMOKE	☐ HONEY	☐ MELON
☐ LEATHER	☐ COFFEE	☐ APPLES	☐ CITRUS
☐ MUSHROOM	☐ MINT	☐ GRASS	☐ OAK
☐ TOBACCO	☐ SPICE	☐ FLORAL	☐ BERRIES
☐ CHOCOLATE	☐ PEPPER	☐ TROPICAL	☐ NUTMEG
☐ JAM	☐ ALMOND	☐ VEGETAL	☐
☐	☐	☐	☐

TASTE

☐ NUTMEG	☐ EARTH	☐ DARK FRUITS	☐ TOAST
☐ VEGETAL	☐ PEPPER	☐ BERRIES	☐ GRASS
☐ FLORAL	☐ VANILLA	☐ PLUMS	☐ CITRUS
☐ HONEY	☐ COFFEE	☐ MUSHROOM	☐ MELON
☐ PEARS	☐ LICORICE	☐ TOBACCO	☐ LYCHE
☐ PEACHES	☐ LEATHER	☐ CHOCOLATE	☐ ALMOND
☐	☐	☐	☐

REVIEW

WINE _____ VINTAGE _____

WHEN _____ WITH _____

WHERE _____ PRICE _____

VARIETAL _____ ALCOHOL (%) _____

BODY   − | | | | | | | +

TANNINS   − | | | | | | | +

SWEETNESS   − | | | | | | | +

INTENSITY   − | | | | | | | +

FINISH   − | | | | | | | +

SMELL

☐ TOAST	☐ SMOKE	☐ HONEY	☐ MELON
☐ LEATHER	☐ COFFEE	☐ APPLES	☐ CITRUS
☐ MUSHROOM	☐ MINT	☐ GRASS	☐ OAK
☐ TOBACCO	☐ SPICE	☐ FLORAL	☐ BERRIES
☐ CHOCOLATE	☐ PEPPER	☐ TROPICAL	☐ NUTMEG
☐ JAM	☐ ALMOND	☐ VEGETAL	☐
☐	☐	☐	☐

TASTE

☐ NUTMEG	☐ EARTH	☐ DARK FRUITS	☐ TOAST
☐ VEGETAL	☐ PEPPER	☐ BERRIES	☐ GRASS
☐ FLORAL	☐ VANILLA	☐ PLUMS	☐ CITRUS
☐ HONEY	☐ COFFEE	☐ MUSHROOM	☐ MELON
☐ PEARS	☐ LICORICE	☐ TOBACCO	☐ LYCHE
☐ PEACHES	☐ LEATHER	☐ CHOCOLATE	☐ ALMOND
☐	☐	☐	☐

REVIEW

WINE _____ VINTAGE _____

WHEN _____ WITH _____

WHERE _____ PRICE _____

VARIETAL _____ ALCOHOL (%) _____

BODY   − | | | | | | | +

TANNINS   − | | | | | | | +

SWEETNESS − | | | | | | | +

INTENSITY − | | | | | | | +

FINISH   − | | | | | | | +

SMELL

- [ ] TOAST
- [ ] LEATHER
- [ ] MUSHROOM
- [ ] TOBACCO
- [ ] CHOCOLATE
- [ ] JAM
- [ ]

- [ ] SMOKE
- [ ] COFFEE
- [ ] MINT
- [ ] SPICE
- [ ] PEPPER
- [ ] ALMOND
- [ ]

- [ ] HONEY
- [ ] APPLES
- [ ] GRASS
- [ ] FLORAL
- [ ] TROPICAL
- [ ] VEGETAL
- [ ]

- [ ] MELON
- [ ] CITRUS
- [ ] OAK
- [ ] BERRIES
- [ ] NUTMEG
- [ ]
- [ ]

TASTE

- [ ] NUTMEG
- [ ] VEGETAL
- [ ] FLORAL
- [ ] HONEY
- [ ] PEARS
- [ ] PEACHES
- [ ]

- [ ] EARTH
- [ ] PEPPER
- [ ] VANILLA
- [ ] COFFEE
- [ ] LICORICE
- [ ] LEATHER
- [ ]

- [ ] DARK FRUITS
- [ ] BERRIES
- [ ] PLUMS
- [ ] MUSHROOM
- [ ] TOBACCO
- [ ] CHOCOLATE
- [ ]

- [ ] TOAST
- [ ] GRASS
- [ ] CITRUS
- [ ] MELON
- [ ] LYCHE
- [ ] ALMOND
- [ ]

WINE		VINTAGE

WHEN		WITH

WHERE		PRICE

VARIETAL		ALCOHOL (%)

BODY   − ☐☐☐☐☐☐ +

TANNINS   − ☐☐☐☐☐☐ +

SWEETNESS   − ☐☐☐☐☐☐ +

INTENSITY   − ☐☐☐☐☐☐ +

FINISH   − ☐☐☐☐☐☐ +

SMELL

☐ TOAST	☐ SMOKE	☐ HONEY	☐ MELON
☐ LEATHER	☐ COFFEE	☐ APPLES	☐ CITRUS
☐ MUSHROOM	☐ MINT	☐ GRASS	☐ OAK
☐ TOBACCO	☐ SPICE	☐ FLORAL	☐ BERRIES
☐ CHOCOLATE	☐ PEPPER	☐ TROPICAL	☐ NUTMEG
☐ JAM	☐ ALMOND	☐ VEGETAL	☐
☐	☐	☐	☐

TASTE

☐ NUTMEG	☐ EARTH	☐ DARK FRUITS	☐ TOAST
☐ VEGETAL	☐ PEPPER	☐ BERRIES	☐ GRASS
☐ FLORAL	☐ VANILLA	☐ PLUMS	☐ CITRUS
☐ HONEY	☐ COFFEE	☐ MUSHROOM	☐ MELON
☐ PEARS	☐ LICORICE	☐ TOBACCO	☐ LYCHE
☐ PEACHES	☐ LEATHER	☐ CHOCOLATE	☐ ALMOND
☐	☐	☐	☐

REVIEW

WINE _____ VINTAGE _____

WHEN _____ WITH _____

WHERE _____ PRICE _____

VARIETAL _____ ALCOHOL (%) _____

BODY   - ☐☐☐☐☐☐ +

TANNINS   - ☐☐☐☐☐☐ +

SWEETNESS - ☐☐☐☐☐☐ +

INTENSITY - ☐☐☐☐☐☐ +

FINISH   - ☐☐☐☐☐☐ +

SMELL

☐ TOAST	☐ SMOKE	☐ HONEY	☐ MELON
☐ LEATHER	☐ COFFEE	☐ APPLES	☐ CITRUS
☐ MUSHROOM	☐ MINT	☐ GRASS	☐ OAK
☐ TOBACCO	☐ SPICE	☐ FLORAL	☐ BERRIES
☐ CHOCOLATE	☐ PEPPER	☐ TROPICAL	☐ NUTMEG
☐ JAM	☐ ALMOND	☐ VEGETAL	☐
☐	☐	☐	☐

TASTE

☐ NUTMEG	☐ EARTH	☐ DARK FRUITS	☐ TOAST
☐ VEGETAL	☐ PEPPER	☐ BERRIES	☐ GRASS
☐ FLORAL	☐ VANILLA	☐ PLUMS	☐ CITRUS
☐ HONEY	☐ COFFEE	☐ MUSHROOM	☐ MELON
☐ PEARS	☐ LICORICE	☐ TOBACCO	☐ LYCHE
☐ PEACHES	☐ LEATHER	☐ CHOCOLATE	☐ ALMOND
☐	☐	☐	☐

REVIEW

RATING

WINE _____ VINTAGE _____

WHEN _____ WITH _____

WHERE _____ PRICE _____

VARIETAL _____ ALCOHOL (%) _____

BODY   − | | | | | | | +

TANNINS   − | | | | | | | +

SWEETNESS − | | | | | | | +

INTENSITY − | | | | | | | +

FINISH   − | | | | | | | +

SMELL

☐ TOAST	☐ SMOKE	☐ HONEY	☐ MELON
☐ LEATHER	☐ COFFEE	☐ APPLES	☐ CITRUS
☐ MUSHROOM	☐ MINT	☐ GRASS	☐ OAK
☐ TOBACCO	☐ SPICE	☐ FLORAL	☐ BERRIES
☐ CHOCOLATE	☐ PEPPER	☐ TROPICAL	☐ NUTMEG
☐ JAM	☐ ALMOND	☐ VEGETAL	☐
☐	☐	☐	☐

TASTE

☐ NUTMEG	☐ EARTH	☐ DARK FRUITS	☐ TOAST
☐ VEGETAL	☐ PEPPER	☐ BERRIES	☐ GRASS
☐ FLORAL	☐ VANILLA	☐ PLUMS	☐ CITRUS
☐ HONEY	☐ COFFEE	☐ MUSHROOM	☐ MELON
☐ PEARS	☐ LICORICE	☐ TOBACCO	☐ LYCHE
☐ PEACHES	☐ LEATHER	☐ CHOCOLATE	☐ ALMOND
☐	☐	☐	☐

REVIEW

RATING

WINE _____   VINTAGE _____

WHEN _____   WITH _____

WHERE _____   PRICE _____

VARIETAL _____   ALCOHOL (%) _____

BODY   - [| | | | |] +

TANNINS   - [| | | | |] +

SWEETNESS - [| | | | |] +

INTENSITY - [| | | | |] +

FINISH   - [| | | | |] +

SMELL

☐ TOAST	☐ SMOKE	☐ HONEY	☐ MELON
☐ LEATHER	☐ COFFEE	☐ APPLES	☐ CITRUS
☐ MUSHROOM	☐ MINT	☐ GRASS	☐ OAK
☐ TOBACCO	☐ SPICE	☐ FLORAL	☐ BERRIES
☐ CHOCOLATE	☐ PEPPER	☐ TROPICAL	☐ NUTMEG
☐ JAM	☐ ALMOND	☐ VEGETAL	☐
☐	☐	☐	☐

TASTE

☐ NUTMEG	☐ EARTH	☐ DARK FRUITS	☐ TOAST
☐ VEGETAL	☐ PEPPER	☐ BERRIES	☐ GRASS
☐ FLORAL	☐ VANILLA	☐ PLUMS	☐ CITRUS
☐ HONEY	☐ COFFEE	☐ MUSHROOM	☐ MELON
☐ PEARS	☐ LICORICE	☐ TOBACCO	☐ LYCHE
☐ PEACHES	☐ LEATHER	☐ CHOCOLATE	☐ ALMOND
☐	☐	☐	☐

REVIEW

RATING

WINE _____ VINTAGE _____

WHEN _____ WITH _____

WHERE _____ PRICE _____

VARIETAL _____ ALCOHOL (%) _____

BODY   - [| | | | |] +

TANNINS   - [| | | | |] +

SWEETNESS - [| | | | |] +

INTENSITY - [| | | | |] +

FINISH   - [| | | | |] +

SMELL

☐ TOAST	☐ SMOKE	☐ HONEY	☐ MELON
☐ LEATHER	☐ COFFEE	☐ APPLES	☐ CITRUS
☐ MUSHROOM	☐ MINT	☐ GRASS	☐ OAK
☐ TOBACCO	☐ SPICE	☐ FLORAL	☐ BERRIES
☐ CHOCOLATE	☐ PEPPER	☐ TROPICAL	☐ NUTMEG
☐ JAM	☐ ALMOND	☐ VEGETAL	☐
☐	☐	☐	☐

TASTE

☐ NUTMEG	☐ EARTH	☐ DARK FRUITS	☐ TOAST
☐ VEGETAL	☐ PEPPER	☐ BERRIES	☐ GRASS
☐ FLORAL	☐ VANILLA	☐ PLUMS	☐ CITRUS
☐ HONEY	☐ COFFEE	☐ MUSHROOM	☐ MELON
☐ PEARS	☐ LICORICE	☐ TOBACCO	☐ LYCHE
☐ PEACHES	☐ LEATHER	☐ CHOCOLATE	☐ ALMOND
☐	☐	☐	☐

REVIEW

RATING

WINE _____ VINTAGE _____

WHEN _____ WITH _____

WHERE _____ PRICE _____

VARIETAL _____ ALCOHOL (%) _____

BODY   – | | | | | | | +

TANNINS   – | | | | | | | +

SWEETNESS – | | | | | | | +

INTENSITY – | | | | | | | +

FINISH   – | | | | | | | +

SMELL

☐ TOAST	☐ SMOKE	☐ HONEY	☐ MELON
☐ LEATHER	☐ COFFEE	☐ APPLES	☐ CITRUS
☐ MUSHROOM	☐ MINT	☐ GRASS	☐ OAK
☐ TOBACCO	☐ SPICE	☐ FLORAL	☐ BERRIES
☐ CHOCOLATE	☐ PEPPER	☐ TROPICAL	☐ NUTMEG
☐ JAM	☐ ALMOND	☐ VEGETAL	☐
☐	☐	☐	☐

TASTE

☐ NUTMEG	☐ EARTH	☐ DARK FRUITS	☐ TOAST
☐ VEGETAL	☐ PEPPER	☐ BERRIES	☐ GRASS
☐ FLORAL	☐ VANILLA	☐ PLUMS	☐ CITRUS
☐ HONEY	☐ COFFEE	☐ MUSHROOM	☐ MELON
☐ PEARS	☐ LICORICE	☐ TOBACCO	☐ LYCHE
☐ PEACHES	☐ LEATHER	☐ CHOCOLATE	☐ ALMOND
☐	☐	☐	☐

REVIEW

RATING

WINE _____ VINTAGE _____

WHEN _____ WITH _____

WHERE _____ PRICE _____

VARIETAL _____ ALCOHOL (%) _____

BODY   - ☐ ☐ ☐ ☐ ☐ ☐ +

TANNINS   - ☐ ☐ ☐ ☐ ☐ ☐ +

SWEETNESS   - ☐ ☐ ☐ ☐ ☐ ☐ +

INTENSITY   - ☐ ☐ ☐ ☐ ☐ ☐ +

FINISH   - ☐ ☐ ☐ ☐ ☐ ☐ +

SMELL

☐ TOAST	☐ SMOKE	☐ HONEY	☐ MELON
☐ LEATHER	☐ COFFEE	☐ APPLES	☐ CITRUS
☐ MUSHROOM	☐ MINT	☐ GRASS	☐ OAK
☐ TOBACCO	☐ SPICE	☐ FLORAL	☐ BERRIES
☐ CHOCOLATE	☐ PEPPER	☐ TROPICAL	☐ NUTMEG
☐ JAM	☐ ALMOND	☐ VEGETAL	
☐	☐	☐	☐

TASTE

☐ NUTMEG	☐ EARTH	☐ DARK FRUITS	☐ TOAST
☐ VEGETAL	☐ PEPPER	☐ BERRIES	☐ GRASS
☐ FLORAL	☐ VANILLA	☐ PLUMS	☐ CITRUS
☐ HONEY	☐ COFFEE	☐ MUSHROOM	☐ MELON
☐ PEARS	☐ LICORICE	☐ TOBACCO	☐ LYCHE
☐ PEACHES	☐ LEATHER	☐ CHOCOLATE	☐ ALMOND
☐	☐	☐	☐

REVIEW

RATING

WINE		VINTAGE	

WHEN	WITH

WHERE	PRICE

VARIETAL	ALCOHOL (%)

BODY   - [| | | | |] +

TANNINS   - [| | | | |] +

SWEETNESS   - [| | | | |] +

INTENSITY   - [| | | | |] +

FINISH   - [| | | | |] +

SMELL

☐ TOAST	☐ SMOKE	☐ HONEY	☐ MELON
☐ LEATHER	☐ COFFEE	☐ APPLES	☐ CITRUS
☐ MUSHROOM	☐ MINT	☐ GRASS	☐ OAK
☐ TOBACCO	☐ SPICE	☐ FLORAL	☐ BERRIES
☐ CHOCOLATE	☐ PEPPER	☐ TROPICAL	☐ NUTMEG
☐ JAM	☐ ALMOND	☐ VEGETAL	☐
☐	☐	☐	☐

TASTE

☐ NUTMEG	☐ EARTH	☐ DARK FRUITS	☐ TOAST
☐ VEGETAL	☐ PEPPER	☐ BERRIES	☐ GRASS
☐ FLORAL	☐ VANILLA	☐ PLUMS	☐ CITRUS
☐ HONEY	☐ COFFEE	☐ MUSHROOM	☐ MELON
☐ PEARS	☐ LICORICE	☐ TOBACCO	☐ LYCHE
☐ PEACHES	☐ LEATHER	☐ CHOCOLATE	☐ ALMOND
☐	☐	☐	☐

REVIEW

RATING

WINE _____ VINTAGE _____

WHEN _____ WITH _____

WHERE _____ PRICE _____

VARIETAL _____ ALCOHOL (%) _____

BODY   − [| | | | |] +

TANNINS   − [| | | | |] +

SWEETNESS   − [| | | | |] +

INTENSITY   − [| | | | |] +

FINISH   − [| | | | |] +

SMELL

☐ TOAST	☐ SMOKE	☐ HONEY	☐ MELON
☐ LEATHER	☐ COFFEE	☐ APPLES	☐ CITRUS
☐ MUSHROOM	☐ MINT	☐ GRASS	☐ OAK
☐ TOBACCO	☐ SPICE	☐ FLORAL	☐ BERRIES
☐ CHOCOLATE	☐ PEPPER	☐ TROPICAL	☐ NUTMEG
☐ JAM	☐ ALMOND	☐ VEGETAL	☐
☐	☐	☐	☐

TASTE

☐ NUTMEG	☐ EARTH	☐ DARK FRUITS	☐ TOAST
☐ VEGETAL	☐ PEPPER	☐ BERRIES	☐ GRASS
☐ FLORAL	☐ VANILLA	☐ PLUMS	☐ CITRUS
☐ HONEY	☐ COFFEE	☐ MUSHROOM	☐ MELON
☐ PEARS	☐ LICORICE	☐ TOBACCO	☐ LYCHE
☐ PEACHES	☐ LEATHER	☐ CHOCOLATE	☐ ALMOND
☐	☐	☐	☐

REVIEW

RATING

WINE _____ VINTAGE _____

WHEN _____ WITH _____

WHERE _____ PRICE _____

VARIETAL _____ ALCOHOL (%) _____

BODY   − | | | | | | | +

TANNINS   − | | | | | | | +

SWEETNESS   − | | | | | | | +

INTENSITY   − | | | | | | | +

FINISH   − | | | | | | | +

SMELL

☐ TOAST	☐ SMOKE	☐ HONEY	☐ MELON
☐ LEATHER	☐ COFFEE	☐ APPLES	☐ CITRUS
☐ MUSHROOM	☐ MINT	☐ GRASS	☐ OAK
☐ TOBACCO	☐ SPICE	☐ FLORAL	☐ BERRIES
☐ CHOCOLATE	☐ PEPPER	☐ TROPICAL	☐ NUTMEG
☐ JAM	☐ ALMOND	☐ VEGETAL	☐
☐	☐	☐	☐

TASTE

☐ NUTMEG	☐ EARTH	☐ DARK FRUITS	☐ TOAST
☐ VEGETAL	☐ PEPPER	☐ BERRIES	☐ GRASS
☐ FLORAL	☐ VANILLA	☐ PLUMS	☐ CITRUS
☐ HONEY	☐ COFFEE	☐ MUSHROOM	☐ MELON
☐ PEARS	☐ LICORICE	☐ TOBACCO	☐ LYCHE
☐ PEACHES	☐ LEATHER	☐ CHOCOLATE	☐ ALMOND
☐	☐	☐	☐

REVIEW

RATING

WINE _____ VINTAGE _____

WHEN _____ WITH _____

WHERE _____ PRICE _____

VARIETAL _____ ALCOHOL (%) _____

BODY   - | | | | | | | +

TANNINS   - | | | | | | | +

SWEETNESS - | | | | | | | +

INTENSITY - | | | | | | | +

FINISH   - | | | | | | | +

SMELL

☐ TOAST	☐ SMOKE	☐ HONEY	☐ MELON
☐ LEATHER	☐ COFFEE	☐ APPLES	☐ CITRUS
☐ MUSHROOM	☐ MINT	☐ GRASS	☐ OAK
☐ TOBACCO	☐ SPICE	☐ FLORAL	☐ BERRIES
☐ CHOCOLATE	☐ PEPPER	☐ TROPICAL	☐ NUTMEG
☐ JAM	☐ ALMOND	☐ VEGETAL	☐
☐	☐	☐	☐

TASTE

☐ NUTMEG	☐ EARTH	☐ DARK FRUITS	☐ TOAST
☐ VEGETAL	☐ PEPPER	☐ BERRIES	☐ GRASS
☐ FLORAL	☐ VANILLA	☐ PLUMS	☐ CITRUS
☐ HONEY	☐ COFFEE	☐ MUSHROOM	☐ MELON
☐ PEARS	☐ LICORICE	☐ TOBACCO	☐ LYCHE
☐ PEACHES	☐ LEATHER	☐ CHOCOLATE	☐ ALMOND
☐	☐	☐	☐

REVIEW

WINE		VINTAGE
WHEN		WITH
WHERE		PRICE
VARIETAL		ALCOHOL (%)

BODY   - ☐☐☐☐☐☐ +

TANNINS   - ☐☐☐☐☐☐ +

SWEETNESS - ☐☐☐☐☐☐ +

INTENSITY - ☐☐☐☐☐☐ +

FINISH   - ☐☐☐☐☐☐ +

SMELL

☐ TOAST	☐ SMOKE	☐ HONEY	☐ MELON
☐ LEATHER	☐ COFFEE	☐ APPLES	☐ CITRUS
☐ MUSHROOM	☐ MINT	☐ GRASS	☐ OAK
☐ TOBACCO	☐ SPICE	☐ FLORAL	☐ BERRIES
☐ CHOCOLATE	☐ PEPPER	☐ TROPICAL	☐ NUTMEG
☐ JAM	☐ ALMOND	☐ VEGETAL	☐
☐	☐	☐	☐

TASTE

☐ NUTMEG	☐ EARTH	☐ DARK FRUITS	☐ TOAST
☐ VEGETAL	☐ PEPPER	☐ BERRIES	☐ GRASS
☐ FLORAL	☐ VANILLA	☐ PLUMS	☐ CITRUS
☐ HONEY	☐ COFFEE	☐ MUSHROOM	☐ MELON
☐ PEARS	☐ LICORICE	☐ TOBACCO	☐ LYCHE
☐ PEACHES	☐ LEATHER	☐ CHOCOLATE	☐ ALMOND
☐	☐	☐	☐

REVIEW

RATING

WINE _____ VINTAGE _____

WHEN _____ WITH _____

WHERE _____ PRICE _____

VARIETAL _____ ALCOHOL (%) _____

BODY   − [| | | | |] +

TANNINS   − [| | | | |] +

SWEETNESS − [| | | | |] +

INTENSITY − [| | | | |] +

FINISH   − [| | | | |] +

SMELL

☐ TOAST	☐ SMOKE	☐ HONEY	☐ MELON
☐ LEATHER	☐ COFFEE	☐ APPLES	☐ CITRUS
☐ MUSHROOM	☐ MINT	☐ GRASS	☐ OAK
☐ TOBACCO	☐ SPICE	☐ FLORAL	☐ BERRIES
☐ CHOCOLATE	☐ PEPPER	☐ TROPICAL	☐ NUTMEG
☐ JAM	☐ ALMOND	☐ VEGETAL	☐
☐	☐	☐	☐

TASTE

☐ NUTMEG	☐ EARTH	☐ DARK FRUITS	☐ TOAST
☐ VEGETAL	☐ PEPPER	☐ BERRIES	☐ GRASS
☐ FLORAL	☐ VANILLA	☐ PLUMS	☐ CITRUS
☐ HONEY	☐ COFFEE	☐ MUSHROOM	☐ MELON
☐ PEARS	☐ LICORICE	☐ TOBACCO	☐ LYCHE
☐ PEACHES	☐ LEATHER	☐ CHOCOLATE	☐ ALMOND
☐	☐	☐	☐

WINE _____   VINTAGE _____

WHEN _____   WITH _____

WHERE _____   PRICE _____

VARIETAL _____   ALCOHOL (%) _____

BODY	−						+
TANNINS	−						+
SWEETNESS	−						+
INTENSITY	−						+
FINISH	−						+

SMELL

☐ TOAST	☐ SMOKE	☐ HONEY	☐ MELON
☐ LEATHER	☐ COFFEE	☐ APPLES	☐ CITRUS
☐ MUSHROOM	☐ MINT	☐ GRASS	☐ OAK
☐ TOBACCO	☐ SPICE	☐ FLORAL	☐ BERRIES
☐ CHOCOLATE	☐ PEPPER	☐ TROPICAL	☐ NUTMEG
☐ JAM	☐ ALMOND	☐ VEGETAL	☐
☐	☐	☐	☐

TASTE

☐ NUTMEG	☐ EARTH	☐ DARK FRUITS	☐ TOAST
☐ VEGETAL	☐ PEPPER	☐ BERRIES	☐ GRASS
☐ FLORAL	☐ VANILLA	☐ PLUMS	☐ CITRUS
☐ HONEY	☐ COFFEE	☐ MUSHROOM	☐ MELON
☐ PEARS	☐ LICORICE	☐ TOBACCO	☐ LYCHE
☐ PEACHES	☐ LEATHER	☐ CHOCOLATE	☐ ALMOND
☐	☐	☐	☐

RATING

WINE _____ VINTAGE _____

WHEN _____ WITH _____

WHERE _____ PRICE _____

VARIETAL _____ ALCOHOL (%) _____

BODY   - [| | | | |] +

TANNINS   - [| | | | |] +

SWEETNESS   - [| | | | |] +

INTENSITY   - [| | | | |] +

FINISH   - [| | | | |] +

SMELL

- [ ] TOAST
- [ ] LEATHER
- [ ] MUSHROOM
- [ ] TOBACCO
- [ ] CHOCOLATE
- [ ] JAM
- [ ]

- [ ] SMOKE
- [ ] COFFEE
- [ ] MINT
- [ ] SPICE
- [ ] PEPPER
- [ ] ALMOND
- [ ]

- [ ] HONEY
- [ ] APPLES
- [ ] GRASS
- [ ] FLORAL
- [ ] TROPICAL
- [ ] VEGETAL
- [ ]

- [ ] MELON
- [ ] CITRUS
- [ ] OAK
- [ ] BERRIES
- [ ] NUTMEG
- [ ]

TASTE

- [ ] NUTMEG
- [ ] VEGETAL
- [ ] FLORAL
- [ ] HONEY
- [ ] PEARS
- [ ] PEACHES
- [ ]

- [ ] EARTH
- [ ] PEPPER
- [ ] VANILLA
- [ ] COFFEE
- [ ] LICORICE
- [ ] LEATHER
- [ ]

- [ ] DARK FRUITS
- [ ] BERRIES
- [ ] PLUMS
- [ ] MUSHROOM
- [ ] TOBACCO
- [ ] CHOCOLATE
- [ ]

- [ ] TOAST
- [ ] GRASS
- [ ] CITRUS
- [ ] MELON
- [ ] LYCHE
- [ ] ALMOND
- [ ]

REVIEW

WINE _____ VINTAGE _____

WHEN _____ WITH _____

WHERE _____ PRICE _____

VARIETAL _____ ALCOHOL (%) _____

BODY   - [ ] [ ] [ ] [ ] [ ] [ ] +

TANNINS   - [ ] [ ] [ ] [ ] [ ] [ ] +

SWEETNESS   - [ ] [ ] [ ] [ ] [ ] [ ] +

INTENSITY   - [ ] [ ] [ ] [ ] [ ] [ ] +

FINISH   - [ ] [ ] [ ] [ ] [ ] [ ] +

SMELL

[ ] TOAST	[ ] SMOKE	[ ] HONEY	[ ] MELON
[ ] LEATHER	[ ] COFFEE	[ ] APPLES	[ ] CITRUS
[ ] MUSHROOM	[ ] MINT	[ ] GRASS	[ ] OAK
[ ] TOBACCO	[ ] SPICE	[ ] FLORAL	[ ] BERRIES
[ ] CHOCOLATE	[ ] PEPPER	[ ] TROPICAL	[ ] NUTMEG
[ ] JAM	[ ] ALMOND	[ ] VEGETAL	[ ]
[ ]	[ ]	[ ]	[ ]

TASTE

[ ] NUTMEG	[ ] EARTH	[ ] DARK FRUITS	[ ] TOAST
[ ] VEGETAL	[ ] PEPPER	[ ] BERRIES	[ ] GRASS
[ ] FLORAL	[ ] VANILLA	[ ] PLUMS	[ ] CITRUS
[ ] HONEY	[ ] COFFEE	[ ] MUSHROOM	[ ] MELON
[ ] PEARS	[ ] LICORICE	[ ] TOBACCO	[ ] LYCHE
[ ] PEACHES	[ ] LEATHER	[ ] CHOCOLATE	[ ] ALMOND
[ ]	[ ]	[ ]	[ ]

REVIEW

RATING

WINE _____ VINTAGE _____

WHEN _____ WITH _____

WHERE _____ PRICE _____

VARIETAL _____ ALCOHOL (%) _____

BODY   - | | | | | | | +

TANNINS   - | | | | | | | +

SWEETNESS   - | | | | | | | +

INTENSITY   - | | | | | | | +

FINISH   - | | | | | | | +

SMELL

- [ ] TOAST
- [ ] LEATHER
- [ ] MUSHROOM
- [ ] TOBACCO
- [ ] CHOCOLATE
- [ ] JAM
- [ ]

- [ ] SMOKE
- [ ] COFFEE
- [ ] MINT
- [ ] SPICE
- [ ] PEPPER
- [ ] ALMOND
- [ ]

- [ ] HONEY
- [ ] APPLES
- [ ] GRASS
- [ ] FLORAL
- [ ] TROPICAL
- [ ] VEGETAL
- [ ]

- [ ] MELON
- [ ] CITRUS
- [ ] OAK
- [ ] BERRIES
- [ ] NUTMEG
- [ ]

TASTE

- [ ] NUTMEG
- [ ] VEGETAL
- [ ] FLORAL
- [ ] HONEY
- [ ] PEARS
- [ ] PEACHES
- [ ]

- [ ] EARTH
- [ ] PEPPER
- [ ] VANILLA
- [ ] COFFEE
- [ ] LICORICE
- [ ] LEATHER
- [ ]

- [ ] DARK FRUITS
- [ ] BERRIES
- [ ] PLUMS
- [ ] MUSHROOM
- [ ] TOBACCO
- [ ] CHOCOLATE
- [ ]

- [ ] TOAST
- [ ] GRASS
- [ ] CITRUS
- [ ] MELON
- [ ] LYCHE
- [ ] ALMOND

REVIEW

RATING

WINE _____ VINTAGE _____

WHEN _____ WITH _____

WHERE _____ PRICE _____

VARIETAL _____ ALCOHOL (%) _____

BODY   − | | | | | | | +

TANNINS   − | | | | | | | +

SWEETNESS   − | | | | | | | +

INTENSITY   − | | | | | | | +

FINISH   − | | | | | | | +

SMELL

☐ TOAST	☐ SMOKE	☐ HONEY	☐ MELON
☐ LEATHER	☐ COFFEE	☐ APPLES	☐ CITRUS
☐ MUSHROOM	☐ MINT	☐ GRASS	☐ OAK
☐ TOBACCO	☐ SPICE	☐ FLORAL	☐ BERRIES
☐ CHOCOLATE	☐ PEPPER	☐ TROPICAL	☐ NUTMEG
☐ JAM	☐ ALMOND	☐ VEGETAL	☐
☐	☐	☐	☐

TASTE

☐ NUTMEG	☐ EARTH	☐ DARK FRUITS	☐ TOAST
☐ VEGETAL	☐ PEPPER	☐ BERRIES	☐ GRASS
☐ FLORAL	☐ VANILLA	☐ PLUMS	☐ CITRUS
☐ HONEY	☐ COFFEE	☐ MUSHROOM	☐ MELON
☐ PEARS	☐ LICORICE	☐ TOBACCO	☐ LYCHE
☐ PEACHES	☐ LEATHER	☐ CHOCOLATE	☐ ALMOND
☐	☐	☐	☐

REVIEW

RATING

WINE _____ VINTAGE _____

WHEN _____ WITH _____

WHERE _____ PRICE _____

VARIETAL _____ ALCOHOL (%) _____

BODY   - | | | | | | | +

TANNINS   - | | | | | | | +

SWEETNESS - | | | | | | | +

INTENSITY - | | | | | | | +

FINISH   - | | | | | | | +

SMELL

☐ TOAST	☐ SMOKE	☐ HONEY	☐ MELON
☐ LEATHER	☐ COFFEE	☐ APPLES	☐ CITRUS
☐ MUSHROOM	☐ MINT	☐ GRASS	☐ OAK
☐ TOBACCO	☐ SPICE	☐ FLORAL	☐ BERRIES
☐ CHOCOLATE	☐ PEPPER	☐ TROPICAL	☐ NUTMEG
☐ JAM	☐ ALMOND	☐ VEGETAL	☐
☐	☐	☐	☐

TASTE

☐ NUTMEG	☐ EARTH	☐ DARK FRUITS	☐ TOAST
☐ VEGETAL	☐ PEPPER	☐ BERRIES	☐ GRASS
☐ FLORAL	☐ VANILLA	☐ PLUMS	☐ CITRUS
☐ HONEY	☐ COFFEE	☐ MUSHROOM	☐ MELON
☐ PEARS	☐ LICORICE	☐ TOBACCO	☐ LYCHE
☐ PEACHES	☐ LEATHER	☐ CHOCOLATE	☐ ALMOND
☐	☐	☐	☐

REVIEW

RATING

WINE _____ VINTAGE _____

WHEN _____ WITH _____

WHERE _____ PRICE _____

VARIETAL _____ ALCOHOL (%) _____

BODY   - [| | | | |] +

TANNINS   - [| | | | |] +

SWEETNESS - [| | | | |] +

INTENSITY - [| | | | |] +

FINISH   - [| | | | |] +

SMELL

☐ TOAST	☐ SMOKE	☐ HONEY	☐ MELON
☐ LEATHER	☐ COFFEE	☐ APPLES	☐ CITRUS
☐ MUSHROOM	☐ MINT	☐ GRASS	☐ OAK
☐ TOBACCO	☐ SPICE	☐ FLORAL	☐ BERRIES
☐ CHOCOLATE	☐ PEPPER	☐ TROPICAL	☐ NUTMEG
☐ JAM	☐ ALMOND	☐ VEGETAL	☐
☐	☐	☐	☐

TASTE

☐ NUTMEG	☐ EARTH	☐ DARK FRUITS	☐ TOAST
☐ VEGETAL	☐ PEPPER	☐ BERRIES	☐ GRASS
☐ FLORAL	☐ VANILLA	☐ PLUMS	☐ CITRUS
☐ HONEY	☐ COFFEE	☐ MUSHROOM	☐ MELON
☐ PEARS	☐ LICORICE	☐ TOBACCO	☐ LYCHE
☐ PEACHES	☐ LEATHER	☐ CHOCOLATE	☐ ALMOND
☐	☐	☐	☐

REVIEW

RATING

WINE _____ VINTAGE _____

WHEN _____ WITH _____

WHERE _____ PRICE _____

VARIETAL _____ ALCOHOL (%) _____

BODY   - | | | | | | | +

TANNINS   - | | | | | | | +

SWEETNESS - | | | | | | | +

INTENSITY - | | | | | | | +

FINISH   - | | | | | | | +

SMELL

☐ TOAST	☐ SMOKE	☐ HONEY	☐ MELON
☐ LEATHER	☐ COFFEE	☐ APPLES	☐ CITRUS
☐ MUSHROOM	☐ MINT	☐ GRASS	☐ OAK
☐ TOBACCO	☐ SPICE	☐ FLORAL	☐ BERRIES
☐ CHOCOLATE	☐ PEPPER	☐ TROPICAL	☐ NUTMEG
☐ JAM	☐ ALMOND	☐ VEGETAL	☐
☐	☐	☐	☐

TASTE

☐ NUTMEG	☐ EARTH	☐ DARK FRUITS	☐ TOAST
☐ VEGETAL	☐ PEPPER	☐ BERRIES	☐ GRASS
☐ FLORAL	☐ VANILLA	☐ PLUMS	☐ CITRUS
☐ HONEY	☐ COFFEE	☐ MUSHROOM	☐ MELON
☐ PEARS	☐ LICORICE	☐ TOBACCO	☐ LYCHE
☐ PEACHES	☐ LEATHER	☐ CHOCOLATE	☐ ALMOND
☐	☐	☐	☐

REVIEW

RATING

WINE _____ VINTAGE _____

WHEN _____ WITH _____

WHERE _____ PRICE _____

VARIETAL _____ ALCOHOL (%) _____

BODY － ☐☐☐☐☐☐ ＋

TANNINS － ☐☐☐☐☐☐ ＋

SWEETNESS － ☐☐☐☐☐☐ ＋

INTENSITY － ☐☐☐☐☐☐ ＋

FINISH － ☐☐☐☐☐☐ ＋

SMELL

☐ TOAST ☐ SMOKE ☐ HONEY ☐ MELON
☐ LEATHER ☐ COFFEE ☐ APPLES ☐ CITRUS
☐ MUSHROOM ☐ MINT ☐ GRASS ☐ OAK
☐ TOBACCO ☐ SPICE ☐ FLORAL ☐ BERRIES
☐ CHOCOLATE ☐ PEPPER ☐ TROPICAL ☐ NUTMEG
☐ JAM ☐ ALMOND ☐ VEGETAL ☐
☐ ☐ ☐ ☐

TASTE

☐ NUTMEG ☐ EARTH ☐ DARK FRUITS ☐ TOAST
☐ VEGETAL ☐ PEPPER ☐ BERRIES ☐ GRASS
☐ FLORAL ☐ VANILLA ☐ PLUMS ☐ CITRUS
☐ HONEY ☐ COFFEE ☐ MUSHROOM ☐ MELON
☐ PEARS ☐ LICORICE ☐ TOBACCO ☐ LYCHE
☐ PEACHES ☐ LEATHER ☐ CHOCOLATE ☐ ALMOND
☐ ☐ ☐ ☐

REVIEW

RATING

WINE _____   VINTAGE _____

WHEN _____   WITH _____

WHERE _____   PRICE _____

VARIETAL _____   ALCOHOL (%) _____

BODY   - □□□□□□ +

TANNINS   - □□□□□□ +

SWEETNESS - □□□□□□ +

INTENSITY - □□□□□□ +

FINISH   - □□□□□□ +

SMELL

☐ TOAST	☐ SMOKE	☐ HONEY	☐ MELON
☐ LEATHER	☐ COFFEE	☐ APPLES	☐ CITRUS
☐ MUSHROOM	☐ MINT	☐ GRASS	☐ OAK
☐ TOBACCO	☐ SPICE	☐ FLORAL	☐ BERRIES
☐ CHOCOLATE	☐ PEPPER	☐ TROPICAL	☐ NUTMEG
☐ JAM	☐ ALMOND	☐ VEGETAL	
☐	☐	☐	☐

TASTE

☐ NUTMEG	☐ EARTH	☐ DARK FRUITS	☐ TOAST
☐ VEGETAL	☐ PEPPER	☐ BERRIES	☐ GRASS
☐ FLORAL	☐ VANILLA	☐ PLUMS	☐ CITRUS
☐ HONEY	☐ COFFEE	☐ MUSHROOM	☐ MELON
☐ PEARS	☐ LICORICE	☐ TOBACCO	☐ LYCHE
☐ PEACHES	☐ LEATHER	☐ CHOCOLATE	☐ ALMOND
☐	☐	☐	☐

REVIEW

RATING

WINE _____ VINTAGE _____

WHEN _____ WITH _____

WHERE _____ PRICE _____

VARIETAL _____ ALCOHOL (%) _____

BODY   − [| | | | |] +

TANNINS   − [| | | | |] +

SWEETNESS   − [| | | | |] +

INTENSITY   − [| | | | |] +

FINISH   − [| | | | |] +

SMELL

☐ TOAST	☐ SMOKE	☐ HONEY	☐ MELON
☐ LEATHER	☐ COFFEE	☐ APPLES	☐ CITRUS
☐ MUSHROOM	☐ MINT	☐ GRASS	☐ OAK
☐ TOBACCO	☐ SPICE	☐ FLORAL	☐ BERRIES
☐ CHOCOLATE	☐ PEPPER	☐ TROPICAL	☐ NUTMEG
☐ JAM	☐ ALMOND	☐ VEGETAL	☐
☐	☐	☐	☐

TASTE

☐ NUTMEG	☐ EARTH	☐ DARK FRUITS	☐ TOAST
☐ VEGETAL	☐ PEPPER	☐ BERRIES	☐ GRASS
☐ FLORAL	☐ VANILLA	☐ PLUMS	☐ CITRUS
☐ HONEY	☐ COFFEE	☐ MUSHROOM	☐ MELON
☐ PEARS	☐ LICORICE	☐ TOBACCO	☐ LYCHE
☐ PEACHES	☐ LEATHER	☐ CHOCOLATE	☐ ALMOND
☐	☐	☐	☐

REVIEW

RATING

WINE _____ VINTAGE _____

WHEN _____ WITH _____

WHERE _____ PRICE _____

VARIETAL _____ ALCOHOL (%) _____

BODY   − | | | | | | | +

TANNINS   − | | | | | | | +

SWEETNESS   − | | | | | | | +

INTENSITY   − | | | | | | | +

FINISH   − | | | | | | | +

SMELL

☐ TOAST	☐ SMOKE	☐ HONEY	☐ MELON
☐ LEATHER	☐ COFFEE	☐ APPLES	☐ CITRUS
☐ MUSHROOM	☐ MINT	☐ GRASS	☐ OAK
☐ TOBACCO	☐ SPICE	☐ FLORAL	☐ BERRIES
☐ CHOCOLATE	☐ PEPPER	☐ TROPICAL	☐ NUTMEG
☐ JAM	☐ ALMOND	☐ VEGETAL	☐
☐	☐	☐	☐

TASTE

☐ NUTMEG	☐ EARTH	☐ DARK FRUITS	☐ TOAST
☐ VEGETAL	☐ PEPPER	☐ BERRIES	☐ GRASS
☐ FLORAL	☐ VANILLA	☐ PLUMS	☐ CITRUS
☐ HONEY	☐ COFFEE	☐ MUSHROOM	☐ MELON
☐ PEARS	☐ LICORICE	☐ TOBACCO	☐ LYCHE
☐ PEACHES	☐ LEATHER	☐ CHOCOLATE	☐ ALMOND
☐	☐	☐	☐

REVIEW

RATING

WINE _____ VINTAGE _____

WHEN _____ WITH _____

WHERE _____ PRICE _____

VARIETAL _____ ALCOHOL (%) _____

BODY   - ☐ ☐ ☐ ☐ ☐ ☐ +

TANNINS   - ☐ ☐ ☐ ☐ ☐ ☐ +

SWEETNESS - ☐ ☐ ☐ ☐ ☐ ☐ +

INTENSITY - ☐ ☐ ☐ ☐ ☐ ☐ +

FINISH   - ☐ ☐ ☐ ☐ ☐ ☐ +

SMELL

☐ TOAST	☐ SMOKE	☐ HONEY	☐ MELON
☐ LEATHER	☐ COFFEE	☐ APPLES	☐ CITRUS
☐ MUSHROOM	☐ MINT	☐ GRASS	☐ OAK
☐ TOBACCO	☐ SPICE	☐ FLORAL	☐ BERRIES
☐ CHOCOLATE	☐ PEPPER	☐ TROPICAL	☐ NUTMEG
☐ JAM	☐ ALMOND	☐ VEGETAL	☐
☐	☐	☐	☐

TASTE

☐ NUTMEG	☐ EARTH	☐ DARK FRUITS	☐ TOAST
☐ VEGETAL	☐ PEPPER	☐ BERRIES	☐ GRASS
☐ FLORAL	☐ VANILLA	☐ PLUMS	☐ CITRUS
☐ HONEY	☐ COFFEE	☐ MUSHROOM	☐ MELON
☐ PEARS	☐ LICORICE	☐ TOBACCO	☐ LYCHE
☐ PEACHES	☐ LEATHER	☐ CHOCOLATE	☐ ALMOND
☐	☐	☐	☐

REVIEW

RATING

WINE _____ VINTAGE _____

WHEN _____ WITH _____

WHERE _____ PRICE _____

VARIETAL _____ ALCOHOL (%) _____

BODY   − | | | | | | | +

TANNINS   − | | | | | | | +

SWEETNESS   − | | | | | | | +

INTENSITY   − | | | | | | | +

FINISH   − | | | | | | | +

SMELL

☐ TOAST	☐ SMOKE	☐ HONEY	☐ MELON
☐ LEATHER	☐ COFFEE	☐ APPLES	☐ CITRUS
☐ MUSHROOM	☐ MINT	☐ GRASS	☐ OAK
☐ TOBACCO	☐ SPICE	☐ FLORAL	☐ BERRIES
☐ CHOCOLATE	☐ PEPPER	☐ TROPICAL	☐ NUTMEG
☐ JAM	☐ ALMOND	☐ VEGETAL	☐
☐	☐	☐	☐

TASTE

☐ NUTMEG	☐ EARTH	☐ DARK FRUITS	☐ TOAST
☐ VEGETAL	☐ PEPPER	☐ BERRIES	☐ GRASS
☐ FLORAL	☐ VANILLA	☐ PLUMS	☐ CITRUS
☐ HONEY	☐ COFFEE	☐ MUSHROOM	☐ MELON
☐ PEARS	☐ LICORICE	☐ TOBACCO	☐ LYCHE
☐ PEACHES	☐ LEATHER	☐ CHOCOLATE	☐ ALMOND
☐	☐	☐	☐

RATING

WINE _____ VINTAGE _____

WHEN _____ WITH _____

WHERE _____ PRICE _____

VARIETAL _____ ALCOHOL (%) _____

BODY   - | | | | | | | +

TANNINS   - | | | | | | | +

SWEETNESS - | | | | | | | +

INTENSITY - | | | | | | | +

FINISH   - | | | | | | | +

SMELL

☐ TOAST	☐ SMOKE	☐ HONEY	☐ MELON
☐ LEATHER	☐ COFFEE	☐ APPLES	☐ CITRUS
☐ MUSHROOM	☐ MINT	☐ GRASS	☐ OAK
☐ TOBACCO	☐ SPICE	☐ FLORAL	☐ BERRIES
☐ CHOCOLATE	☐ PEPPER	☐ TROPICAL	☐ NUTMEG
☐ JAM	☐ ALMOND	☐ VEGETAL	☐
☐	☐	☐	☐

TASTE

☐ NUTMEG	☐ EARTH	☐ DARK FRUITS	☐ TOAST
☐ VEGETAL	☐ PEPPER	☐ BERRIES	☐ GRASS
☐ FLORAL	☐ VANILLA	☐ PLUMS	☐ CITRUS
☐ HONEY	☐ COFFEE	☐ MUSHROOM	☐ MELON
☐ PEARS	☐ LICORICE	☐ TOBACCO	☐ LYCHE
☐ PEACHES	☐ LEATHER	☐ CHOCOLATE	☐ ALMOND
☐	☐	☐	☐

REVIEW

RATING

WINE _____ VINTAGE _____

WHEN _____ WITH _____

WHERE _____ PRICE _____

VARIETAL _____ ALCOHOL (%) _____

BODY   - [ ][ ][ ][ ][ ][ ] +

TANNINS   - [ ][ ][ ][ ][ ][ ] +

SWEETNESS   - [ ][ ][ ][ ][ ][ ] +

INTENSITY   - [ ][ ][ ][ ][ ][ ] +

FINISH   - [ ][ ][ ][ ][ ][ ] +

SMELL

[ ] TOAST	[ ] SMOKE	[ ] HONEY	[ ] MELON
[ ] LEATHER	[ ] COFFEE	[ ] APPLES	[ ] CITRUS
[ ] MUSHROOM	[ ] MINT	[ ] GRASS	[ ] OAK
[ ] TOBACCO	[ ] SPICE	[ ] FLORAL	[ ] BERRIES
[ ] CHOCOLATE	[ ] PEPPER	[ ] TROPICAL	[ ] NUTMEG
[ ] JAM	[ ] ALMOND	[ ] VEGETAL	[ ]
[ ]	[ ]	[ ]	[ ]

TASTE

[ ] NUTMEG	[ ] EARTH	[ ] DARK FRUITS	[ ] TOAST
[ ] VEGETAL	[ ] PEPPER	[ ] BERRIES	[ ] GRASS
[ ] FLORAL	[ ] VANILLA	[ ] PLUMS	[ ] CITRUS
[ ] HONEY	[ ] COFFEE	[ ] MUSHROOM	[ ] MELON
[ ] PEARS	[ ] LICORICE	[ ] TOBACCO	[ ] LYCHE
[ ] PEACHES	[ ] LEATHER	[ ] CHOCOLATE	[ ] ALMOND
[ ]	[ ]	[ ]	[ ]

REVIEW

RATING

WINE _____ VINTAGE _____

WHEN _____ WITH _____

WHERE _____ PRICE _____

VARIETAL _____ ALCOHOL (%) _____

BODY   − | | | | | | | +

TANNINS   − | | | | | | | +

SWEETNESS   − | | | | | | | +

INTENSITY   − | | | | | | | +

FINISH   − | | | | | | | +

SMELL

☐ TOAST	☐ SMOKE	☐ HONEY	☐ MELON
☐ LEATHER	☐ COFFEE	☐ APPLES	☐ CITRUS
☐ MUSHROOM	☐ MINT	☐ GRASS	☐ OAK
☐ TOBACCO	☐ SPICE	☐ FLORAL	☐ BERRIES
☐ CHOCOLATE	☐ PEPPER	☐ TROPICAL	☐ NUTMEG
☐ JAM	☐ ALMOND	☐ VEGETAL	☐
☐	☐	☐	☐

TASTE

☐ NUTMEG	☐ EARTH	☐ DARK FRUITS	☐ TOAST
☐ VEGETAL	☐ PEPPER	☐ BERRIES	☐ GRASS
☐ FLORAL	☐ VANILLA	☐ PLUMS	☐ CITRUS
☐ HONEY	☐ COFFEE	☐ MUSHROOM	☐ MELON
☐ PEARS	☐ LICORICE	☐ TOBACCO	☐ LYCHE
☐ PEACHES	☐ LEATHER	☐ CHOCOLATE	☐ ALMOND
☐	☐	☐	☐

REVIEW

RATING

WINE _____ VINTAGE _____

WHEN _____ WITH _____

WHERE _____ PRICE _____

VARIETAL _____ ALCOHOL (%) _____

BODY   - | | | | | | | +

TANNINS   - | | | | | | | +

SWEETNESS   - | | | | | | | +

INTENSITY   - | | | | | | | +

FINISH   - | | | | | | | +

SMELL

- [ ] TOAST
- [ ] LEATHER
- [ ] MUSHROOM
- [ ] TOBACCO
- [ ] CHOCOLATE
- [ ] JAM
- [ ]

- [ ] SMOKE
- [ ] COFFEE
- [ ] MINT
- [ ] SPICE
- [ ] PEPPER
- [ ] ALMOND
- [ ]

- [ ] HONEY
- [ ] APPLES
- [ ] GRASS
- [ ] FLORAL
- [ ] TROPICAL
- [ ] VEGETAL
- [ ]

- [ ] MELON
- [ ] CITRUS
- [ ] OAK
- [ ] BERRIES
- [ ] NUTMEG
- [ ]

TASTE

- [ ] NUTMEG
- [ ] VEGETAL
- [ ] FLORAL
- [ ] HONEY
- [ ] PEARS
- [ ] PEACHES
- [ ]

- [ ] EARTH
- [ ] PEPPER
- [ ] VANILLA
- [ ] COFFEE
- [ ] LICORICE
- [ ] LEATHER
- [ ]

- [ ] DARK FRUITS
- [ ] BERRIES
- [ ] PLUMS
- [ ] MUSHROOM
- [ ] TOBACCO
- [ ] CHOCOLATE
- [ ]

- [ ] TOAST
- [ ] GRASS
- [ ] CITRUS
- [ ] MELON
- [ ] LYCHE
- [ ] ALMOND
- [ ]

WINE _____ VINTAGE _____

WHEN _____ WITH _____

WHERE _____ PRICE _____

VARIETAL _____ ALCOHOL (%) _____

BODY   - ☐ ☐ ☐ ☐ ☐ ☐ +

TANNINS   - ☐ ☐ ☐ ☐ ☐ ☐ +

SWEETNESS - ☐ ☐ ☐ ☐ ☐ ☐ +

INTENSITY - ☐ ☐ ☐ ☐ ☐ ☐ +

FINISH   - ☐ ☐ ☐ ☐ ☐ ☐ +

SMELL

☐ TOAST	☐ SMOKE	☐ HONEY	☐ MELON
☐ LEATHER	☐ COFFEE	☐ APPLES	☐ CITRUS
☐ MUSHROOM	☐ MINT	☐ GRASS	☐ OAK
☐ TOBACCO	☐ SPICE	☐ FLORAL	☐ BERRIES
☐ CHOCOLATE	☐ PEPPER	☐ TROPICAL	☐ NUTMEG
☐ JAM	☐ ALMOND	☐ VEGETAL	☐
☐	☐	☐	☐

TASTE

☐ NUTMEG	☐ EARTH	☐ DARK FRUITS	☐ TOAST
☐ VEGETAL	☐ PEPPER	☐ BERRIES	☐ GRASS
☐ FLORAL	☐ VANILLA	☐ PLUMS	☐ CITRUS
☐ HONEY	☐ COFFEE	☐ MUSHROOM	☐ MELON
☐ PEARS	☐ LICORICE	☐ TOBACCO	☐ LYCHE
☐ PEACHES	☐ LEATHER	☐ CHOCOLATE	☐ ALMOND
☐	☐	☐	☐

REVIEW

RATING

WINE _____   VINTAGE _____

WHEN _____   WITH _____

WHERE _____   PRICE _____

VARIETAL _____   ALCOHOL (%) _____

BODY   - [| | | | |] +

TANNINS   - [| | | | |] +

SWEETNESS - [| | | | |] +

INTENSITY - [| | | | |] +

FINISH   - [| | | | |] +

SMELL

- [ ] TOAST
- [ ] LEATHER
- [ ] MUSHROOM
- [ ] TOBACCO
- [ ] CHOCOLATE
- [ ] JAM
- [ ]

- [ ] SMOKE
- [ ] COFFEE
- [ ] MINT
- [ ] SPICE
- [ ] PEPPER
- [ ] ALMOND
- [ ]

- [ ] HONEY
- [ ] APPLES
- [ ] GRASS
- [ ] FLORAL
- [ ] TROPICAL
- [ ] VEGETAL
- [ ]

- [ ] MELON
- [ ] CITRUS
- [ ] OAK
- [ ] BERRIES
- [ ] NUTMEG
- [ ]

TASTE

- [ ] NUTMEG
- [ ] VEGETAL
- [ ] FLORAL
- [ ] HONEY
- [ ] PEARS
- [ ] PEACHES
- [ ]

- [ ] EARTH
- [ ] PEPPER
- [ ] VANILLA
- [ ] COFFEE
- [ ] LICORICE
- [ ] LEATHER
- [ ]

- [ ] DARK FRUITS
- [ ] BERRIES
- [ ] PLUMS
- [ ] MUSHROOM
- [ ] TOBACCO
- [ ] CHOCOLATE
- [ ]

- [ ] TOAST
- [ ] GRASS
- [ ] CITRUS
- [ ] MELON
- [ ] LYCHE
- [ ] ALMOND
- [ ]

REVIEW

RATING

WINE _____ VINTAGE _____

WHEN _____ WITH _____

WHERE _____ PRICE _____

VARIETAL _____ ALCOHOL (%) _____

BODY − ☐☐☐☐☐☐ +

TANNINS − ☐☐☐☐☐☐ +

SWEETNESS − ☐☐☐☐☐☐ +

INTENSITY − ☐☐☐☐☐☐ +

FINISH − ☐☐☐☐☐☐ +

SMELL

☐ TOAST	☐ SMOKE	☐ HONEY	☐ MELON
☐ LEATHER	☐ COFFEE	☐ APPLES	☐ CITRUS
☐ MUSHROOM	☐ MINT	☐ GRASS	☐ OAK
☐ TOBACCO	☐ SPICE	☐ FLORAL	☐ BERRIES
☐ CHOCOLATE	☐ PEPPER	☐ TROPICAL	☐ NUTMEG
☐ JAM	☐ ALMOND	☐ VEGETAL	☐
☐	☐	☐	☐

TASTE

☐ NUTMEG	☐ EARTH	☐ DARK FRUITS	☐ TOAST
☐ VEGETAL	☐ PEPPER	☐ BERRIES	☐ GRASS
☐ FLORAL	☐ VANILLA	☐ PLUMS	☐ CITRUS
☐ HONEY	☐ COFFEE	☐ MUSHROOM	☐ MELON
☐ PEARS	☐ LICORICE	☐ TOBACCO	☐ LYCHE
☐ PEACHES	☐ LEATHER	☐ CHOCOLATE	☐ ALMOND
☐	☐	☐	☐

REVIEW

RATING

WINE _____ VINTAGE _____

WHEN _____ WITH _____

WHERE _____ PRICE _____

VARIETAL _____ ALCOHOL (%) _____

BODY   - | | | | | | | +

TANNINS   - | | | | | | | +

SWEETNESS   - | | | | | | | +

INTENSITY   - | | | | | | | +

FINISH   - | | | | | | | +

SMELL

- [ ] TOAST
- [ ] LEATHER
- [ ] MUSHROOM
- [ ] TOBACCO
- [ ] CHOCOLATE
- [ ] JAM
- [ ]

- [ ] SMOKE
- [ ] COFFEE
- [ ] MINT
- [ ] SPICE
- [ ] PEPPER
- [ ] ALMOND
- [ ]

- [ ] HONEY
- [ ] APPLES
- [ ] GRASS
- [ ] FLORAL
- [ ] TROPICAL
- [ ] VEGETAL
- [ ]

- [ ] MELON
- [ ] CITRUS
- [ ] OAK
- [ ] BERRIES
- [ ] NUTMEG
- [ ]

TASTE

- [ ] NUTMEG
- [ ] VEGETAL
- [ ] FLORAL
- [ ] HONEY
- [ ] PEARS
- [ ] PEACHES
- [ ]

- [ ] EARTH
- [ ] PEPPER
- [ ] VANILLA
- [ ] COFFEE
- [ ] LICORICE
- [ ] LEATHER
- [ ]

- [ ] DARK FRUITS
- [ ] BERRIES
- [ ] PLUMS
- [ ] MUSHROOM
- [ ] TOBACCO
- [ ] CHOCOLATE
- [ ]

- [ ] TOAST
- [ ] GRASS
- [ ] CITRUS
- [ ] MELON
- [ ] LYCHE
- [ ] ALMOND
- [ ]

REVIEW

RATING

WINE _____ VINTAGE _____

WHEN _____ WITH _____

WHERE _____ PRICE _____

VARIETAL _____ ALCOHOL (%) _____

BODY   − | | | | | | | +

TANNINS   − | | | | | | | +

SWEETNESS   − | | | | | | | +

INTENSITY   − | | | | | | | +

FINISH   − | | | | | | | +

SMELL

- [ ] TOAST
- [ ] LEATHER
- [ ] MUSHROOM
- [ ] TOBACCO
- [ ] CHOCOLATE
- [ ] JAM
- [ ]

- [ ] SMOKE
- [ ] COFFEE
- [ ] MINT
- [ ] SPICE
- [ ] PEPPER
- [ ] ALMOND
- [ ]

- [ ] HONEY
- [ ] APPLES
- [ ] GRASS
- [ ] FLORAL
- [ ] TROPICAL
- [ ] VEGETAL
- [ ]

- [ ] MELON
- [ ] CITRUS
- [ ] OAK
- [ ] BERRIES
- [ ] NUTMEG
- [ ]

TASTE

- [ ] NUTMEG
- [ ] VEGETAL
- [ ] FLORAL
- [ ] HONEY
- [ ] PEARS
- [ ] PEACHES
- [ ]

- [ ] EARTH
- [ ] PEPPER
- [ ] VANILLA
- [ ] COFFEE
- [ ] LICORICE
- [ ] LEATHER
- [ ]

- [ ] DARK FRUITS
- [ ] BERRIES
- [ ] PLUMS
- [ ] MUSHROOM
- [ ] TOBACCO
- [ ] CHOCOLATE
- [ ]

- [ ] TOAST
- [ ] GRASS
- [ ] CITRUS
- [ ] MELON
- [ ] LYCHE
- [ ] ALMOND

WINE _____ VINTAGE _____

WHEN _____ WITH _____

WHERE _____ PRICE _____

VARIETAL _____ ALCOHOL (%) _____

BODY   - [ ][ ][ ][ ][ ][ ] +

TANNINS   - [ ][ ][ ][ ][ ][ ] +

SWEETNESS - [ ][ ][ ][ ][ ][ ] +

INTENSITY - [ ][ ][ ][ ][ ][ ] +

FINISH   - [ ][ ][ ][ ][ ][ ] +

SMELL

☐ TOAST	☐ SMOKE	☐ HONEY	☐ MELON
☐ LEATHER	☐ COFFEE	☐ APPLES	☐ CITRUS
☐ MUSHROOM	☐ MINT	☐ GRASS	☐ OAK
☐ TOBACCO	☐ SPICE	☐ FLORAL	☐ BERRIES
☐ CHOCOLATE	☐ PEPPER	☐ TROPICAL	☐ NUTMEG
☐ JAM	☐ ALMOND	☐ VEGETAL	☐
☐	☐	☐	☐

TASTE

☐ NUTMEG	☐ EARTH	☐ DARK FRUITS	☐ TOAST
☐ VEGETAL	☐ PEPPER	☐ BERRIES	☐ GRASS
☐ FLORAL	☐ VANILLA	☐ PLUMS	☐ CITRUS
☐ HONEY	☐ COFFEE	☐ MUSHROOM	☐ MELON
☐ PEARS	☐ LICORICE	☐ TOBACCO	☐ LYCHE
☐ PEACHES	☐ LEATHER	☐ CHOCOLATE	☐ ALMOND
☐	☐	☐	☐

RATING

WINE _____   VINTAGE _____

WHEN _____   WITH _____

WHERE _____   PRICE _____

VARIETAL _____   ALCOHOL (%) _____

BODY   − [ ][ ][ ][ ][ ][ ] +

TANNINS   − [ ][ ][ ][ ][ ][ ] +

SWEETNESS   − [ ][ ][ ][ ][ ][ ] +

INTENSITY   − [ ][ ][ ][ ][ ][ ] +

FINISH   − [ ][ ][ ][ ][ ][ ] +

SMELL

☐ TOAST	☐ SMOKE	☐ HONEY	☐ MELON
☐ LEATHER	☐ COFFEE	☐ APPLES	☐ CITRUS
☐ MUSHROOM	☐ MINT	☐ GRASS	☐ OAK
☐ TOBACCO	☐ SPICE	☐ FLORAL	☐ BERRIES
☐ CHOCOLATE	☐ PEPPER	☐ TROPICAL	☐ NUTMEG
☐ JAM	☐ ALMOND	☐ VEGETAL	☐
☐	☐	☐	☐

TASTE

☐ NUTMEG	☐ EARTH	☐ DARK FRUITS	☐ TOAST
☐ VEGETAL	☐ PEPPER	☐ BERRIES	☐ GRASS
☐ FLORAL	☐ VANILLA	☐ PLUMS	☐ CITRUS
☐ HONEY	☐ COFFEE	☐ MUSHROOM	☐ MELON
☐ PEARS	☐ LICORICE	☐ TOBACCO	☐ LYCHE
☐ PEACHES	☐ LEATHER	☐ CHOCOLATE	☐ ALMOND
☐	☐	☐	☐

REVIEW

RATING

WINE _____ VINTAGE _____

WHEN _____ WITH _____

WHERE _____ PRICE _____

VARIETAL _____ ALCOHOL (%) _____

BODY   - | | | | | | | +

TANNINS   - | | | | | | | +

SWEETNESS   - | | | | | | | +

INTENSITY   - | | | | | | | +

FINISH   - | | | | | | | +

SMELL

- [ ] TOAST
- [ ] LEATHER
- [ ] MUSHROOM
- [ ] TOBACCO
- [ ] CHOCOLATE
- [ ] JAM
- [ ]

- [ ] SMOKE
- [ ] COFFEE
- [ ] MINT
- [ ] SPICE
- [ ] PEPPER
- [ ] ALMOND
- [ ]

- [ ] HONEY
- [ ] APPLES
- [ ] GRASS
- [ ] FLORAL
- [ ] TROPICAL
- [ ] VEGETAL
- [ ]

- [ ] MELON
- [ ] CITRUS
- [ ] OAK
- [ ] BERRIES
- [ ] NUTMEG
- [ ]

TASTE

- [ ] NUTMEG
- [ ] VEGETAL
- [ ] FLORAL
- [ ] HONEY
- [ ] PEARS
- [ ] PEACHES
- [ ]

- [ ] EARTH
- [ ] PEPPER
- [ ] VANILLA
- [ ] COFFEE
- [ ] LICORICE
- [ ] LEATHER
- [ ]

- [ ] DARK FRUITS
- [ ] BERRIES
- [ ] PLUMS
- [ ] MUSHROOM
- [ ] TOBACCO
- [ ] CHOCOLATE
- [ ]

- [ ] TOAST
- [ ] GRASS
- [ ] CITRUS
- [ ] MELON
- [ ] LYCHE
- [ ] ALMOND
- [ ]

REVIEW

RATING

WINE _____ VINTAGE _____

WHEN _____ WITH _____

WHERE _____ PRICE _____

VARIETAL _____ ALCOHOL (%) _____

BODY   − ☐☐☐☐☐☐ +

TANNINS   − ☐☐☐☐☐☐ +

SWEETNESS − ☐☐☐☐☐☐ +

INTENSITY − ☐☐☐☐☐☐ +

FINISH   − ☐☐☐☐☐☐ +

SMELL

☐ TOAST	☐ SMOKE	☐ HONEY	☐ MELON
☐ LEATHER	☐ COFFEE	☐ APPLES	☐ CITRUS
☐ MUSHROOM	☐ MINT	☐ GRASS	☐ OAK
☐ TOBACCO	☐ SPICE	☐ FLORAL	☐ BERRIES
☐ CHOCOLATE	☐ PEPPER	☐ TROPICAL	☐ NUTMEG
☐ JAM	☐ ALMOND	☐ VEGETAL	☐
☐	☐	☐	☐

TASTE

☐ NUTMEG	☐ EARTH	☐ DARK FRUITS	☐ TOAST
☐ VEGETAL	☐ PEPPER	☐ BERRIES	☐ GRASS
☐ FLORAL	☐ VANILLA	☐ PLUMS	☐ CITRUS
☐ HONEY	☐ COFFEE	☐ MUSHROOM	☐ MELON
☐ PEARS	☐ LICORICE	☐ TOBACCO	☐ LYCHE
☐ PEACHES	☐ LEATHER	☐ CHOCOLATE	☐ ALMOND
☐	☐	☐	☐

REVIEW

RATING

WINE _____ VINTAGE _____

WHEN _____ WITH _____

WHERE _____ PRICE _____

VARIETAL _____ ALCOHOL (%) _____

BODY   - [| | | | |] +

TANNINS   - [| | | | |] +

SWEETNESS - [| | | | |] +

INTENSITY - [| | | | |] +

FINISH   - [| | | | |] +

SMELL

☐ TOAST	☐ SMOKE	☐ HONEY	☐ MELON
☐ LEATHER	☐ COFFEE	☐ APPLES	☐ CITRUS
☐ MUSHROOM	☐ MINT	☐ GRASS	☐ OAK
☐ TOBACCO	☐ SPICE	☐ FLORAL	☐ BERRIES
☐ CHOCOLATE	☐ PEPPER	☐ TROPICAL	☐ NUTMEG
☐ JAM	☐ ALMOND	☐ VEGETAL	☐
☐	☐	☐	☐

TASTE

☐ NUTMEG	☐ EARTH	☐ DARK FRUITS	☐ TOAST
☐ VEGETAL	☐ PEPPER	☐ BERRIES	☐ GRASS
☐ FLORAL	☐ VANILLA	☐ PLUMS	☐ CITRUS
☐ HONEY	☐ COFFEE	☐ MUSHROOM	☐ MELON
☐ PEARS	☐ LICORICE	☐ TOBACCO	☐ LYCHE
☐ PEACHES	☐ LEATHER	☐ CHOCOLATE	☐ ALMOND
☐	☐	☐	☐

REVIEW

RATING

WINE _____ VINTAGE _____

WHEN _____ WITH _____

WHERE _____ PRICE _____

VARIETAL _____ ALCOHOL (%) _____

BODY   - [| | | | |] +

TANNINS   - [| | | | |] +

SWEETNESS   - [| | | | |] +

INTENSITY   - [| | | | |] +

FINISH   - [| | | | |] +

SMELL

☐ TOAST	☐ SMOKE	☐ HONEY	☐ MELON
☐ LEATHER	☐ COFFEE	☐ APPLES	☐ CITRUS
☐ MUSHROOM	☐ MINT	☐ GRASS	☐ OAK
☐ TOBACCO	☐ SPICE	☐ FLORAL	☐ BERRIES
☐ CHOCOLATE	☐ PEPPER	☐ TROPICAL	☐ NUTMEG
☐ JAM	☐ ALMOND	☐ VEGETAL	☐
☐	☐	☐	☐

TASTE

☐ NUTMEG	☐ EARTH	☐ DARK FRUITS	☐ TOAST
☐ VEGETAL	☐ PEPPER	☐ BERRIES	☐ GRASS
☐ FLORAL	☐ VANILLA	☐ PLUMS	☐ CITRUS
☐ HONEY	☐ COFFEE	☐ MUSHROOM	☐ MELON
☐ PEARS	☐ LICORICE	☐ TOBACCO	☐ LYCHE
☐ PEACHES	☐ LEATHER	☐ CHOCOLATE	☐ ALMOND
☐	☐	☐	☐

WINE _____ VINTAGE _____

WHEN _____ WITH _____

WHERE _____ PRICE _____

VARIETAL _____ ALCOHOL (%) _____

BODY   − □□□□□□ +

TANNINS   − □□□□□□ +

SWEETNESS   − □□□□□□ +

INTENSITY   − □□□□□□ +

FINISH   − □□□□□□ +

SMELL

☐ TOAST	☐ SMOKE	☐ HONEY	☐ MELON
☐ LEATHER	☐ COFFEE	☐ APPLES	☐ CITRUS
☐ MUSHROOM	☐ MINT	☐ GRASS	☐ OAK
☐ TOBACCO	☐ SPICE	☐ FLORAL	☐ BERRIES
☐ CHOCOLATE	☐ PEPPER	☐ TROPICAL	☐ NUTMEG
☐ JAM	☐ ALMOND	☐ VEGETAL	☐
☐	☐	☐	☐

TASTE

☐ NUTMEG	☐ EARTH	☐ DARK FRUITS	☐ TOAST
☐ VEGETAL	☐ PEPPER	☐ BERRIES	☐ GRASS
☐ FLORAL	☐ VANILLA	☐ PLUMS	☐ CITRUS
☐ HONEY	☐ COFFEE	☐ MUSHROOM	☐ MELON
☐ PEARS	☐ LICORICE	☐ TOBACCO	☐ LYCHE
☐ PEACHES	☐ LEATHER	☐ CHOCOLATE	☐ ALMOND
☐	☐	☐	☐

REVIEW

RATING

WINE _____ VINTAGE _____

WHEN _____ WITH _____

WHERE _____ PRICE _____

VARIETAL _____ ALCOHOL (%) _____

BODY   − ☐ ☐ ☐ ☐ ☐ ☐ +

TANNINS   − ☐ ☐ ☐ ☐ ☐ ☐ +

SWEETNESS   − ☐ ☐ ☐ ☐ ☐ ☐ +

INTENSITY   − ☐ ☐ ☐ ☐ ☐ ☐ +

FINISH   − ☐ ☐ ☐ ☐ ☐ ☐ +

SMELL

☐ TOAST	☐ SMOKE	☐ HONEY	☐ MELON
☐ LEATHER	☐ COFFEE	☐ APPLES	☐ CITRUS
☐ MUSHROOM	☐ MINT	☐ GRASS	☐ OAK
☐ TOBACCO	☐ SPICE	☐ FLORAL	☐ BERRIES
☐ CHOCOLATE	☐ PEPPER	☐ TROPICAL	☐ NUTMEG
☐ JAM	☐ ALMOND	☐ VEGETAL	☐
☐	☐	☐	☐

TASTE

☐ NUTMEG	☐ EARTH	☐ DARK FRUITS	☐ TOAST
☐ VEGETAL	☐ PEPPER	☐ BERRIES	☐ GRASS
☐ FLORAL	☐ VANILLA	☐ PLUMS	☐ CITRUS
☐ HONEY	☐ COFFEE	☐ MUSHROOM	☐ MELON
☐ PEARS	☐ LICORICE	☐ TOBACCO	☐ LYCHE
☐ PEACHES	☐ LEATHER	☐ CHOCOLATE	☐ ALMOND
☐	☐	☐	☐

Made in the USA
Las Vegas, NV
17 April 2023